Intermittent fasting for women over 40.

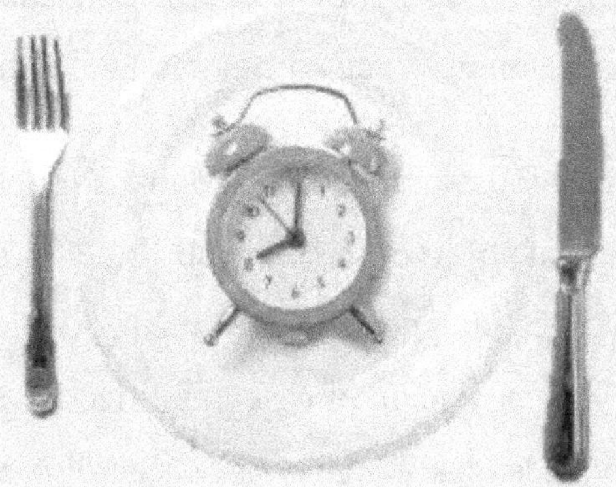

The Comprehensive Guide to Gut Health, Weight Loss, Hormonal Balance, and Menopause with Delectable RecipeS.

Dr Marcia Moss

Copyright © 2023 by Dr Marcia Moss.

The information provided in this book is for educational purposes and is not intended as a substitute for professional medical advice, diagnosis, or treatment. Always seek the advice of your physician or other qualified health provider with any questions you may have regarding a medical condition

Thank You for Choosing Our Book

We understand that embarking on your journey to a healthier diet is a significant commitment, and we want to support you every step of the way. As a token of our appreciation for choosing this book. we're thrilled to offer you a special incentive.

Free Consultation for Book Purchasers

For those who have purchased the book, we're delighted to extend a free consultation to address any specific questions, concerns, or guidance you may need on your path to healthy intermittent fasting. Our team of experts is here to provide you with personalized advice to make your journey as smooth and effective as possible. This consultation is exclusively available to book purchasers, and we're eager to assist you in achieving your goals. To access the free consultation, simply reach out to us at

drmarciamoss@gmail.com

OTHER BOOKS BY THE AUTHOR

1. Insulin Resistance Diet for Weight Loss: *The Complete Guide to Managing Insulin Resistance and Achieving Your Weight Loss Goals*

Aligning with the weight management aspect of your intermittent fasting book, this title offers a comprehensive guide to addressing insulin resistance for effective weight loss.

2. Colitis Relief Juicing: *A Comprehensive Guide to Soothing Your Gut: Over 30 Nutrient-Packed Recipes for Managing Colitis Symptoms and Restoring Digestive Health Naturally*

With a focus on digestive health, this book complements the gut wellness element in your intermittent fasting guide, providing practical solutions for managing colitis symptoms.

Table of Contents

A Journey of Transformation

Meet Jane, a vibrant woman in her 40s, juggling the demands of family, work, and the ever-elusive quest for personal well-being. Like many of us, Jane found herself at a crossroads, feeling the weight of time on her shoulders and yearning for a change that felt sustainable and, most importantly, hers.

As Jane embarked on her journey into the world of intermittent fasting, she wasn't seeking a quick fix or a temporary solution. Instead, she sought a path that would harmonize with the rhythm of her life—a rhythm uniquely tuned to the needs of a woman navigating the exciting and, at times, challenging terrain of her 40s.

The beauty of Jane's story lies not in a dramatic overnight transformation but in the gradual, empowering shifts that occurred. She discovered that intermittent fasting was not just a dietary strategy but a holistic approach that resonated with the ebb and flow of her daily existence.

In the pages ahead, you will not find complex theories or unreachable goals. This is not a book about strict regimens or one-size-fits-all solutions. It's a companion for those who understand that life is a journey, not a race, and that well-being is a continuous, evolving process.

As you delve into the insights and wisdom shared within, envision Jane's story as a beacon of reassurance. Imagine her discovering newfound energy, experiencing the joy of balanced meals, and reclaiming control over her health. This book is not just about intermittent fasting; it's about acknowledging the power you hold to make sustainable choices and carve a path that aligns with your unique journey.

So, dear reader, as you turn the pages, let the stories of real women guide you, let the practical advice empower you, and let the reassurance within these words echo: You are indeed at the right place—a place where health meets wisdom, where simplicity triumphs over complexity, and where your journey towards well-being begins. Welcome to a narrative that embraces you, uplifts you, and celebrates the remarkable woman you are.

Introduction

Ever thought your digestive system deserves a vacation? That's intermittent fasting in a nutshell.

What is Intermittent Fasting?

At its core, Intermittent Fasting is not a complex puzzle. It's not about forbidden foods or an elaborate set of rules that demand a degree in nutrition to decipher. In simple terms, it's a way of structuring your meals and the time you spend eating. Instead of a constant flow of snacks and meals throughout the day, you'll be embracing cycles of eating and fasting.

Now, you might be thinking, "Why change the way I've been eating for years?" That's a fair question, and the answer lies in the remarkable benefits that Intermittent Fasting holds, especially for women navigating the journey beyond 40.

Why Intermittent Fasting for Women Over 40?

As we gracefully age, our bodies undergo subtle transformations. Metabolism may slow down, hormonal shifts become more pronounced, and the quest for maintaining a healthy weight can feel like an uphill battle. This is where Intermittent Fasting steps in as a companion in your health journey.

For women over 40, IF offers a tailored approach to weight management, acknowledging the unique aspects of your body's changes. It's not a one-size-fits-all solution but a flexible strategy that adapts to your lifestyle, providing a sustainable path toward well-being.

Benefits and Misconceptions

Let's clear the air on a few fronts. The benefits of Intermittent Fasting extend beyond weight management. Scientifically backed, it has shown promise in enhancing cognitive function, promoting cellular repair, and even contributing to longevity. It's not just about shedding pounds; it's about embracing a holistic approach to health.

However, amidst the genuine benefits, a few misconceptions often float around. Some may argue that skipping meals is detrimental, but Intermittent Fasting is not about deprivation. It's about creating a rhythm that aligns with your body's natural cycles, allowing it to function optimally.

Chapter 1: The Basics of Intermittent Fasting

Understanding Different IF Protocols

Let's break down the different ways you can embrace intermittent fasting. Think of these as tools in your health toolkit, each with its own unique approach.

1. 16/8 Method: Your Daily Routine Transformer

Ever heard of the 16/8 method? It's like giving your body a daily reset button. For 16 hours, your stomach takes a break, and during the remaining 8 hours, you feast (within reason, of course). This method seamlessly integrates into your daily routine, letting you eat when it suits you.

2. 5:2 Diet: Embracing the Power of Flexibility

The 5:2 diet is like a part-time gig for your stomach. For two non-consecutive days, you dial down your calorie intake, giving your body a chance to recalibrate. On the other five days, you eat your regular meals without counting every morsel. It's a flexible approach that doesn't feel like a perpetual diet, making it an excellent fit for the dynamic lifestyle of women over 40.

3. Alternate-Day Fasting: Intermittent Breaks for Your Body

Alternate-day fasting takes the intermittent game up a notch. One day you eat as you normally would, and the next, you cut back. It's a bit like a seesaw, giving your body a break every other day. Simple, right?

4. Time-Restricted Eating: A Clockwork Approach

Time-restricted eating is all about setting a clock for your meals. You choose a specific window for eating, and outside of that, your stomach clock is on pause. It's not about counting calories or overthinking – just aligning your meals with the natural rhythm of the day.

Now, why bother with these methods? Well, they aren't some secret code to unlock a mystical health realm, but rather tools to make intermittent fasting work for you. They offer flexibility, allowing you to pick what suits your lifestyle and preferences.

Choosing Your Fasting Path

The beauty of intermittent fasting lies in its adaptability. You're not locked into a one-size-fits-all plan. Instead, you can choose the approach that fits seamlessly into your life, making it a sustainable and enjoyable journey.

As we move forward in this book, we'll explore how these methods can be customized to your unique needs.Remember, this is about simplicity, not complexity.

Chapter 2: Tailoring Intermittent Fasting for Women Over 40

In this chapter, we'll explore how intermittent fasting (IF) can be tailored to harmonize with the changes women experience during this stage of life.

Hormonal Changes and IF

For many women over 40, hormonal changes become more pronounced, often accompanied by shifts in metabolism. Intermittent fasting can be a helpful ally during this time. As our bodies adjust, insulin sensitivity may change, affecting how we process sugars and store fat. IF, with its rhythmic eating and fasting cycles, has shown promise in regulating insulin levels.

Oestrogen is an important part of the hormone symphony. As oestrogen levels fluctuate during pre-menopause and menopause, women may experience weight gain and changes in fat distribution. IF can be a powerful tool to manage these changes by promoting fat utilization for energy during fasting periods.

Addressing Menopausal Challenges

Menopause is a part of life many women navigate with resilience and grace. Yet, it brings its own set of challenges, from hot flashes to changes in metabolism. Intermittent fasting can be a gentle guide through these challenges.

One of the perks of IF during menopause lies in its potential to support weight management. As metabolism tends to slow down, adopting an IF routine can help kickstart fat burning and maintain muscle mass. Moreover, IF has been linked to improvements in insulin sensitivity, offering a natural ally against the insulin resistance that sometimes accompanies menopause.

In this journey, it's crucial to approach IF with a compassionate mindset. The goal isn't to impose strict rules but to create a sustainable and adaptable framework that aligns with your body's evolving needs. Embrace the flexibility inherent in IF, allowing it to complement your unique menopausal experience.

Adapting IF to Your Lifestyle

Now, let's address the practical side of things – integrating IF into your daily life. The beauty of IF is its versatility, making it accessible for various lifestyles and preferences. Whether you're a morning person or a night owl, there's a way to tailor IF to suit you.

Begin by considering your daily routine and personal preferences. If breakfast is your favourite meal, the 16/8 method might be your ally, allowing you to enjoy a hearty morning meal and compress your eating window later in the day. On the other hand, if dinner gatherings are your social sanctuary, an early time-restricted eating window might be the perfect fit.

Chapter 3: Mastering Weight Management

Embarking on the journey of intermittent fasting (IF) holds a unique promise for women over 40, a promise that extends beyond mere weight loss. In this chapter, we'll navigate the science behind weight management with IF, explore the foundations of a sustainable exercise routine, and tackle the metabolic slowdown that often accompanies the passage of time.

The Science of Weight Loss and IF

Intermittent fasting isn't a magic trick; it's a science-backed approach to weight management that aligns with the body's natural rhythms. For women over

40, understanding this science is key to unlocking the full potential of IF.

As we age, our metabolism undergoes changes, and shedding those extra pounds becomes more challenging. IF, however, offers a strategic ally in this battle. By embracing designated eating windows and periods of fasting, the body taps into stored fat for energy, promoting weight loss without sacrificing muscle mass.

It's crucial to approach IF not as a restrictive diet but as a lifestyle shift. By allowing the body to experience periods of nourishment and rest, women over 40 can cultivate a sustainable weight management strategy that goes beyond the numbers on the scale.

Building a Sustainable Exercise Routine

While IF lays a solid foundation for weight management, the synergy with a well-designed exercise routine is unparalleled. The goal isn't just to shed pounds but to enhance overall health and well-being.

Consider incorporating a mix of cardiovascular exercises, strength training, and flexibility exercises into your routine. This trifecta addresses not only weight loss but also bone density, muscle mass, and joint health—key concerns for women navigating the intricacies of the fourth decade and beyond.

Engaging in activities you enjoy is paramount. Whether it's a brisk walk, a dance class, or yoga in the living room, finding joy in movement ensures long-term adherence. Moreover, exercising with friends or family can transform physical activity into a social experience, adding an extra layer of motivation and accountability.

Combating Metabolic Slowdown

Metabolism isn't a constant; it evolves over time, and for women over 40, this evolution may mean a metabolic slowdown. The good news is that IF has shown promise in mitigating this natural progression.

Intermittent fasting prompts the body to become more metabolically flexible, adapting to changing energy demands efficiently. This flexibility counteracts the tendency to store excess calories as fat, a common occurrence in the face of a slowing metabolism.

Incorporating metabolism-boosting foods, such as lean proteins, whole grains, and vibrant vegetables, complements the efforts of IF. These nutrient-dense choices not only support weight management but also contribute to overall health and vitality.

In conclusion, mastering weight management with intermittent fasting involves embracing the science behind it, crafting a sustainable exercise routine, and addressing the nuances of metabolic changes. This journey is not just about shedding pounds; it's about reclaiming control over one's well-being and embracing a lifestyle that fosters lasting health.

Chapter 4: Soothing Stomach Woes

Taking care of your stomach becomes even more crucial as you gracefully step into your forties. In this chapter, we'll navigate the terrain of gut health, tackling digestion concerns, and discovering how Intermittent Fasting (IF) can be seamlessly integrated into a gut-friendly lifestyle.

Unravelling the Importance of Gut Health and Digestion

Your gut, often referred to as the body's second brain, plays a pivotal role in overall well-being. As we age, maintaining a healthy gut becomes essential, influencing everything from nutrient absorption to immune function. Intermittent

Fasting, surprisingly simple yet effective, can become your ally in this journey.

IF offers your digestive system a well-deserved break, allowing it to reset and function optimally. During fasting periods, the gut has time to repair and rejuvenate, contributing to improved digestion and nutrient assimilation. It's like giving your digestive system a reset button, promoting a healthier gut environment.

Navigating Digestive Discomfort with Intermittent Fasting

Digestive discomfort is a common companion, especially as the years add up. The good news is that Intermittent Fasting can be a gentle balm for an upset stomach. By giving your digestive system scheduled breaks, IF reduces the overall load on your gut, easing common discomforts like bloating and indigestion.

This approach isn't about stringent dietary restrictions. It's a simple, adaptable strategy that allows your digestive system the space and time it needs to process food efficiently. As a woman over 40, embracing IF may mean finding relief from the digestive woes that have become all too familiar.

Harmonizing IF with a Gut-Friendly Diet

IF, when harmoniously paired with a gut-friendly diet, can be a game-changer for women in their forties. So, what does a gut-friendly diet look like?

Firstly, consider incorporating fiber-rich foods into your meals. Vegetables, fruits, and whole grains not only support digestion but also nourish the beneficial bacteria in your gut. These friendly bacteria play a crucial role in maintaining a balanced gut environment.

Secondly, stay hydrated. Water is a simple yet powerful elixir for your gut. It helps in the smooth passage of food through your digestive system and ensures your gut remains adequately lubricated.

Lastly, be mindful of processed foods. Opt for whole, unprocessed options that are easier on your digestive system. IF, coupled with a diet rich in these elements, creates a synergy that promotes a healthier and happier gut.

Chapter 6: Delectable IF Recipes for Women Over 40

Breakfast Delights

Energizing Smoothies

Recipe 1: Berry Bliss Smoothie

Ingredients:

- 1 cup mixed berries (strawberries, blueberries, raspberries)

- 1 banana

- 1/2 cup Greek yogurt

- 1 tablespoon chia seeds

- 1 cup almond milk

Instructions:

1. Blend mixed berries, banana, and Greek yogurt until smooth.

2. Add chia seeds and almond milk, blend again until well combined.

3. Pour into a glass and enjoy this antioxidant-packed energy booster.

Recipe 2: Tropical Sunrise Smoothie

Ingredients:

- 1/2 cup pineapple chunks

- 1/2 cup mango chunks

- 1/2 banana

- 1/2 cup coconut water

- 1/2 cup orange juice

Instructions:

1. Combine pineapple, mango, banana, coconut water, and orange juice in a blender.

2. Blend until smooth and pour into a tall glass for a taste of the tropics to kickstart your day.

Recipe 3: Green Goddess Smoothie

Ingredients:

- 1 cup spinach leaves

- 1/2 cucumber, peeled and sliced

- 1/2 avocado

- 1/2 lime, juiced

- 1 cup coconut water

Instructions:

1. Blend spinach, cucumber, avocado, lime juice, and coconut water until creamy.

2. Pour into a glass, and revel in the refreshing green goodness.

Recipe 4: Chocolate Almond Joy Smoothie

Ingredients:

- 1 banana

- 2 tablespoons cocoa powder

- 1 tablespoon almond butter

- 1 cup almond milk

- Ice cubes (optional)

Instructions:

1. Blend banana, cocoa powder, almond butter, and almond milk until smooth.

2. Add ice cubes if desired, blend again, and savor the guilt-free pleasure of chocolate and almonds.

Recipe 5: Oatmeal Cookie Smoothie

Ingredients:

- 1/2 cup rolled oats

- 1/2 apple, cored and chopped

- 1/2 teaspoon cinnamon

- 1 tablespoon honey

- 1 cup milk (dairy or plant-based)

Instructions:

1. Blend rolled oats, apple, cinnamon, honey, and milk until oats are well incorporated.

2. Pour into a glass and relish the comforting flavours reminiscent of an oatmeal cookie.

Recipe 6: Coffee Banana Smoothie

Ingredients:

- 1/2 cup brewed coffee, cooled

- 1 banana

- 1/2 cup Greek yogurt

- 1 tablespoon honey

- Ice cubes (optional)

Instructions:

1. Blend brewed coffee, banana, Greek yogurt, and honey until smooth.

2. Add ice cubes if desired for a refreshing and caffeinated start to your morning.

Recipe 7: Veggie-Packed Egg Muffins

Ingredients:

- 4 large eggs

- 1/2 cup of diced bell peppers (any colour)

- 1/2 cup diced tomatoes

- 1/4 cup chopped spinach

- Salt and pepper to taste

Instructions:

1. Preheat your oven to 350°F (175°C) and grease a muffin tin.

2. In a bowl, whisk the eggs and season them with salt and pepper.

3. Stir in bell peppers, tomatoes, and spinach.

4. Pour the mixture into muffin cups and bake for 15-20 minutes or until eggs are set. Enjoy these protein-packed muffins.

Recipe 8: Quinoa Breakfast Bowl

Ingredients:

- 1/2 cup cooked quinoa

- 1/4 cup sliced almonds

- 1/2 cup mixed berries (strawberries, blueberries)

- 1 tablespoon honey

- 1/2 cup Greek yogurt

Instructions:

1. In a bowl, combine cooked quinoa, sliced almonds, and mixed berries.

2. Drizzle honey over the mixture and top with Greek yogurt for a hearty and protein-rich breakfast.

Recipe 9: Salmon and Avocado Toast

Ingredients:

- 2 slices whole-grain bread

- 1/2 avocado, mashed

- 2 ounces smoked salmon

- Lemon wedges for garnish

Instructions:

1. Toast the whole-grain bread slices.

2. Spread mashed avocado on each slice.

3. Top with smoked salmon and garnish with a squeeze of lemon for a delicious, protein-packed twist on traditional toast.

Recipe 10: Cottage Cheese Parfait

Ingredients:

- 1/2 cup low-fat cottage cheese

- 1/2 cup granola

- 1/2 cup mixed berries

- 1 tablespoon honey

Instructions:

1. In a glass, layer cottage cheese, granola, and mixed berries.

2. Drizzle honey over the top, creating a satisfying and protein-filled parfait.

Recipe 11: Spinach and Feta Omelette

Ingredients:

- 3 large eggs

- 1 cup fresh spinach leaves

- 2 tablespoons feta cheese, crumbled

- Salt and pepper to taste

Instructions:

1. Whisk eggs in a bowl and season with salt and pepper.

2. In a non-stick skillet, sauté spinach until wilted.

3. Pour whisked eggs over the spinach, add feta, and cook until set. Fold and serve this protein-packed omelette.

Recipe 12: Greek Yogurt and Berry Smoothie Bowl

Ingredients:

- 1 cup Greek yogurt

- 1/2 cup of assorted berries, including strawberries, blueberries, and raspberries.

- 1 tablespoon chia seeds

- 1 tablespoon almond butter

Instructions:

1. In a bowl, layer Greek yogurt.

2. Top with mixed berries, chia seeds, and a dollop of almond butter for a protein-rich and satisfying smoothie bowl.

Satisfying Lunches

Recipe 13: Grilled Chicken and Quinoa Salad

Ingredients:

- 2 cups mixed salad greens

- 1/2 cup cooked quinoa

- 4 ounces grilled chicken breast, sliced

- 1/4 cup cherry tomatoes, halved

- 1/4 cup cucumber, sliced

- Balsamic vinaigrette dressing

Instructions:

1. In a large bowl, combine salad greens, quinoa, grilled chicken, cherry tomatoes, and cucumber.

2. Drizzle with your favorite balsamic vinaigrette dressing and toss for a balanced and hearty salad.

Recipe 14: Avocado and Shrimp Zoodle Bowl

Ingredients:

- 1 zucchini, spiralized

- 4 ounces cooked shrimp

- 1/2 avocado, sliced

- 1/4 cup red bell pepper, thinly sliced

- 2 tablespoons cilantro, chopped

- Lime vinaigrette dressing

Instructions:

1. Arrange spiralized zucchini in a bowl.

2. Top with cooked shrimp, avocado slices, red bell pepper, and cilantro.

3. Drizzle with lime vinaigrette dressing for a refreshing and low-carb salad.

Recipe 15: Chickpea and Greek Salad

Ingredients:

- 1 can (15 ounces) chickpeas, drained and rinsed

- 1 cup cherry tomatoes, halved

- 1/2 cucumber, diced

- 1/4 cup red onion, finely chopped

- 2 tablespoons feta cheese, crumbled

- Greek dressing

Instructions:

1. In a bowl, combine chickpeas, cherry tomatoes, cucumber, red onion, and feta cheese.

2. Toss with your favorite Greek dressing for a protein-packed and flavorful salad.

Recipe 16: Quinoa and Roasted Vegetable Salad

Ingredients:

- 1 cup cooked quinoa

- 1 cup mixed roasted vegetables (zucchini, bell peppers, cherry tomatoes)

- 1/4 cup crumbled goat cheese

- Fresh basil leaves

- Balsamic glaze

Instructions:

1. Mix cooked quinoa with roasted vegetables in a bowl.

2. Top with crumbled goat cheese, fresh basil leaves, and a drizzle of balsamic glaze for a warm and satisfying salad.

Recipe 17: Asian Sesame Chicken Salad

Ingredients:

- 4 cups shredded cabbage and carrots (coleslaw mix)

- 4 ounces grilled chicken, shredded

- 1/4 cup edamame

- 1/4 cup sliced almonds

- Sesame ginger dressing

Instructions:

1. Combine shredded cabbage and carrots with grilled chicken, edamame, and sliced almonds.

2. Toss with sesame ginger dressing for a crunchy and flavorful Asian-inspired salad.

Recipe 18: Caprese Salad with Balsamic Reduction

Ingredients:

- 2 large tomatoes, sliced

- 1 cup fresh mozzarella, sliced

- Fresh basil leaves

- Balsamic reduction

- Olive oil, for drizzling

Instructions:

1. Arrange tomato and mozzarella slices on a plate.

2. Top with fresh basil leaves and drizzle with balsamic reduction and olive oil for a classic and satisfying Caprese salad.

Recipe 19: Mediterranean Chicken Wrap

Ingredients:

- 1 whole-grain wrap

- 4 ounces grilled chicken strips

- 1/4 cup hummus

- 1/2 cup cucumber, thinly sliced

- 1/4 cup Kalamata olives, sliced

- Fresh parsley, chopped

Instructions:

1. Lay out the whole-grain wrap and spread hummus evenly.

2. Place grilled chicken strips, cucumber slices, and Kalamata olives.

3. Sprinkle with fresh parsley, fold, and enjoy this Mediterranean-inspired delight.

Recipe 20: Black Bean and Veggie Burrito Bowl

Ingredients:

- 1 cup cooked brown rice

- 1/2 cup black beans, drained and rinsed

- 1/2 cup corn kernels

- 1/2 cup cherry tomatoes, halved

- Avocado slices

- Salsa verde

Instructions:

1. In a bowl, layer cooked brown rice, black beans, corn, cherry tomatoes, and avocado slices.

2. Top with salsa verde for a satisfying and protein-packed burrito bowl.

Recipe 21: Turkey and Avocado Lettuce Wraps

Ingredients:

- Large lettuce leaves (such as iceberg or romaine)

- 4 ounces turkey slices

- 1/2 avocado, sliced

- 1/4 cup shredded carrots

- Greek yogurt dressing

Instructions:

1. Place turkey slices on large lettuce leaves.

2. Add avocado slices, shredded carrots, and drizzle with Greek yogurt dressing for a light and refreshing wrap.

Recipe 22: Quinoa and Chickpea Power Bowl

Ingredients:

- 1 cup cooked quinoa

- 1/2 cup chickpeas, roasted

- 1/2 cup cherry tomatoes, halved

- 1/4 cup cucumber, diced

- Feta cheese, crumbled

- Lemon tahini dressing

Instructions:

1. Combine cooked quinoa, roasted chickpeas, cherry tomatoes, and cucumber in a bowl.

2. Sprinkle with crumbled feta and drizzle with lemon tahini dressing for a nutrient-packed power bowl.

Recipe 23: Smoked Salmon and Cream Cheese Wrap

Ingredients:

- 1 whole-grain wrap

- 2 ounces smoked salmon

- 2 tablespoons cream cheese

- Cucumber slices

- Red onion, thinly sliced

- Fresh dill, chopped

Instructions:

1. Spread cream cheese on the whole-grain wrap.

2. Layer smoked salmon, cucumber slices, red onion, and sprinkle with fresh dill. Roll it up for a delightful and filling smoked salmon wrap.

Recipe 24: Southwest Chicken Quinoa Bowl

Ingredients:

- 1 cup cooked quinoa

- 4 ounces grilled chicken, diced

- 1/4 cup black beans, drained and rinsed

- 1/4 cup corn kernels

- Avocado slices

- Chipotle lime dressing

Instructions:

1. In a bowl, combine cooked quinoa, diced grilled chicken, black beans, corn, and avocado slices.

2. Drizzle with chipotle lime dressing for a zesty and satisfying Southwest-inspired quinoa bowl.

Nourishing Dinners

Lean Proteins and Healthy Fats

Recipe 25: Baked Lemon Garlic Salmon

Ingredients:

- 1 salmon fillet (6 ounces)

- 1 tablespoon olive oil

- 1 lemon, juiced

- 2 cloves garlic, minced

- Fresh dill, chopped

- Salt and pepper to taste

Instructions:

1. Preheat the oven to 400°F (200°C).

2. Place the salmon fillet on a baking sheet.

3. In a bowl, mix olive oil, lemon juice, minced garlic, and chopped dill.

4. Drizzle the mixture over the salmon and season with salt and pepper.

5. Bake for 15-20 minutes or until the salmon flakes easily with a fork. Enjoy this flavorful and omega-3 rich dinner.

Recipe 26: Grilled Chicken and Quinoa Stuffed Bell Peppers

Ingredients:

- 2 bell peppers, halved and seeds removed

- 8 ounces grilled chicken, shredded

- 1 cup cooked quinoa

- 1/2 cup black beans, drained and rinsed

- 1/2 cup salsa

- Avocado slices for garnish

Instructions:

1. Preheat the grill or oven to medium-high heat.

2. In a bowl, mix shredded grilled chicken, cooked quinoa, black beans, and salsa.

3. Stuff the bell peppers with the mixture and grill or bake for 15-20 minutes.

4. Garnish with avocado slices for a protein-packed and satisfying dinner.

Recipe 27: Turkey and Sweet Potato Skillet

Ingredients:

- 1 pound lean ground turkey

- 2 sweet potatoes, peeled and diced

- 1 cup broccoli florets

- 1 teaspoon cumin

- 1 teaspoon paprika

- Salt and pepper to taste

- Olive oil for cooking

Instructions:

1. In a skillet, heat olive oil over medium heat.

2. Add ground turkey and cook until browned.

3. Add diced sweet potatoes and broccoli to the skillet.

4. Season with paprika, cumin, pepper and salt and Cook until sweet potatoes are tender.

5. Serve this lean protein and nutrient-rich dish for a comforting and nourishing dinner.

Recipe 28: Quinoa-Stuffed Portobello Mushrooms

Ingredients:

- 4 large portobello mushrooms, stems removed

- 1 cup cooked quinoa

- 1/2 cup cherry tomatoes, diced

- 1/4 cup feta cheese, crumbled

- Fresh basil leaves for garnish

Instructions:

1. Preheat the oven to a temperature of 375°F (190°C).

2. Place portobello mushrooms on a baking sheet.

3. In a bowl, mix cooked quinoa, diced cherry tomatoes, and crumbled feta.

4. Stuff the mushrooms with the quinoa mixture and bake for 20-25 minutes.

5. Garnish with fresh basil leaves for a flavorful and protein-packed vegetarian dinner.

Recipe 29: Shrimp and Asparagus Stir-Fry

Ingredients:

- 8 ounces shrimp, peeled and deveined

- 1 bunch asparagus, trimmed and cut into pieces

- 1 tablespoon soy sauce

- 1 tablespoon sesame oil

- 1 teaspoon ginger, minced

- 2 cloves garlic, minced

Instructions:

1. In a wok or skillet, heat sesame oil over medium-high heat.

2. Add shrimp, asparagus, ginger, and garlic. Stir-fry until shrimp are pink and asparagus is tender.

3. Drizzle with soy sauce and toss to coat. Serve this quick and delicious stir-fry for a protein-rich dinner.

Recipe 30: Greek Turkey Meatballs with Tzatziki

Ingredients:

- 1 pound lean ground turkey

- 1/2 cup whole wheat breadcrumbs

- 1/4 cup red onion, finely chopped

- 2 cloves garlic, minced

- 1 teaspoon oregano

- Salt and pepper to taste

- Tzatziki sauce for dipping

Instructions:

1. Preheat the oven to 375°F (190°C).

2. In a bowl, mix ground turkey, breadcrumbs, red onion, garlic, oregano, salt, and pepper.

3. Form the mixture into meatballs and place on a baking sheet.

4. Place in the oven and bake for 20 to 25 minutes, or until fully cooked.

5. Serve with tzatziki sauce for a flavorful and protein-packed dinner.

Recipe 31: Lentil and Vegetable Stew

Ingredients:

- 1 cup dried green lentils, rinsed

- 1 onion, diced

- 2 carrots, peeled and chopped

- 2 celery stalks, chopped

- 3 cloves garlic, minced

- 1 can (14 ounces) diced tomatoes

- 4 cups vegetable broth

- 1 teaspoon cumin

- 1 teaspoon smoked paprika

\- Salt and pepper to taste

\- Fresh parsley for garnish

Instructions:

1. In a large pot, sauté onion, carrots, celery, and garlic until softened.

2. Add lentils, diced tomatoes, vegetable broth, cumin, smoked paprika, salt, and pepper.

3. Simmer for 25-30 minutes or until lentils are tender.

4. Garnish with fresh parsley for a hearty and plant-based stew.

Recipe 32: Sweet Potato and Chickpea Curry

Ingredients:

- 2 sweet potatoes, peeled and diced

- 1 can of chickpeas, 15 ounces in size, drained
  and rinsed.

- 1 onion, finely chopped

- 2 tablespoons curry powder

- 1 can (14 ounces) coconut milk

- 2 cups spinach leaves

- Brown rice for serving

Instructions:

1. In a large pan, sauté sweet potatoes, chickpeas, and onion until slightly browned.

2. Stir in curry powder and pour in coconut milk. Simmer until sweet potatoes are tender.

3. Add spinach and cook until wilted. Serve over brown rice for a flavorful plant-based curry.

Recipe 33: Quinoa-Stuffed Bell Peppers

Ingredients:

- 4 bell peppers, halved and seeds removed

- 1 cup cooked quinoa

- Drain and rinse a 15-ounce can of black beans.

- 1 cup corn kernels

- 1 cup cherry tomatoes, diced

- 1 teaspoon cumin

- 1 teaspoon chili powder

- Guacamole for topping

Instructions:

1. Preheat the oven to 375°F (190°C).

2. In a bowl, mix cooked quinoa, black beans, corn, cherry tomatoes, cumin, and chili powder.

3. Stuff the bell peppers with the quinoa mixture and bake for 25-30 minutes.

4. Top with guacamole for a satisfying and nutritious plant-based dinner.

Recipe 34: Eggplant and Chickpea Tagine

Ingredients:

- 1 large eggplant, diced

- 1 can of chickpeas, 15 ounces in size, drained
  and rinsed.

- 1 onion, finely chopped

- 2 cloves garlic, minced

- 1 can (14 ounces) diced tomatoes

- 1 teaspoon ground cumin

- 1 teaspoon ground coriander

- Fresh cilantro for garnish

Instructions:

1. In a tagine or large pot, sauté eggplant, chickpeas, onion, and garlic until softened.

2. Stir in diced tomatoes, cumin, and coriander. Simmer until flavors meld.

3. Garnish with fresh cilantro for a Moroccan-inspired plant-based delight.

Recipe 35: Spinach and Mushroom Stuffed Acorn Squash

Ingredients:

- 2 acorn squash, halved and seeds removed

- 2 cups spinach leaves

- 1 cup mushrooms, chopped

- 1/2 cup quinoa, cooked

- 1/4 cup nutritional yeast (optional)

- Salt and pepper to taste

Instructions:

1. Preheat the oven temperature to 400°F (200°C).

2. Place acorn squash halves on a baking sheet.

3. In a pan, sauté spinach, mushrooms, and cooked quinoa until spinach wilts.

4. Stuff acorn squash with the mixture. Sprinkle with nutritional yeast, salt, and pepper.

5. Bake for 30-35 minutes or until squash is tender. Enjoy this wholesome and plant-based dinner.

Recipe 36: Black Bean and Vegetable Stir-Fry

Ingredients:

- 1 can (15 ounces) black beans, drained and rinsed

- 2 cups broccoli florets

- 1 red bell pepper, sliced

- 1 cup snow peas

- 2 tablespoons soy sauce

- 1 tablespoon sesame oil

Instructions:

1. In a wok or skillet, heat sesame oil over medium-high heat.

2. Add black beans, broccoli, red bell pepper, and snow peas. Stir-fry until vegetables are tender-crisp.

3. Drizzle with soy sauce and toss to coat. Serve this quick and flavorful plant-based stir-fry.

Sweet Treats

Guilt-Free Desserts & Snacks

Recipe 37: Chocolate Avocado Mousse

Ingredients:

- 2 ripe avocados

- 1/4 cup unsweetened cocoa powder

- 1/4 cup maple syrup

- 1 teaspoon vanilla extract

- A pinch of salt

- Fresh berries for garnish

Instructions:

1. In a blender, combine avocados, cocoa powder, maple syrup, vanilla extract, and a pinch of salt.

2. Blend until smooth and creamy.

3. Chill in the refrigerator for at least 30 minutes.

4. Serve topped with fresh berries for a decadent and guilt-free chocolate mousse.

Recipe 38: Greek Yogurt Parfait

Ingredients:

- 1 cup Greek yogurt

- 1/2 cup mixed berries (blueberries strawberries, raspberries)

- 1/4 cup granola

- 1 tablespoon honey

Instructions:

1. In a glass, layer Greek yogurt, mixed berries, and granola.

2. Drizzle with honey for a satisfying and protein-packed parfait.

Recipe 39: Banana Nut Energy Bites

Ingredients:

- 2 ripe bananas, mashed

- 1 cup rolled oats

- 1/2 cup almond butter

- 1/4 cup chopped nuts (walnuts, almonds)

- 1 teaspoon cinnamon

- 1/4 cup dark chocolate chips

Instructions:

1. In a bowl, mix mashed bananas, rolled oats, almond butter, chopped nuts, and cinnamon.

2. Fold in dark chocolate chips.

3. Form into bite-sized balls and refrigerate for at least 1 hour and enjoy these nutrient-packed energy bites as a guilt-free snack.

Recipe 40: Berry and Yogurt Popsicles

Ingredients:

- 1 cup mixed berries (strawberries, blueberries, raspberries)

- 2 cups Greek yogurt

- 2 tablespoons honey

Instructions:

1. In a blender, puree mixed berries.

2. In a bowl, mix Greek yogurt with honey.

3. Layer berry puree and yogurt in popsicle molds.

4. Freeze for at least 4 hours. Indulge in these refreshing and guilt-free popsicles.

Recipe 41: Almond and Coconut Bliss Balls

Ingredients:

- 1 cup almonds

- 1/2 cup shredded coconut

- 1/4 cup dates, pitted

- 1 tablespoon coconut oil

- A pinch of sea salt

Instructions:

1. In a food processor, blend almonds until finely ground.

2. Add shredded coconut, dates, coconut oil, and a pinch of sea salt. Blend until a sticky mixture forms.

3. Roll into bite-sized bliss balls and refrigerate for 30 minutes and savour as a guilt-free treat.

Chapter 7: Overcoming Challenges and Staying Consistent

Navigating the path of intermittent fasting involves more than just adjusting meal times; it's about creating a sustainable lifestyle that nurtures your well-being.

Common Hurdles in IF:

Embarking on any transformative journey is met with hurdles, and intermittent fasting is no exception. For women over 40, certain challenges may arise due to hormonal shifts, metabolism changes, and lifestyle factors. It's essential to recognize these hurdles and understand that they are part of the process.

1. **1. Hormonal Fluctuations:** Women in their 40s often experience hormonal changes, including fluctuations in estrogen and progesterone. These shifts can impact hunger levels, energy, and mood. Understanding these changes is key to adapting your fasting routine accordingly.

2. **2. Metabolic Adaptation:** As we age, our metabolism tends to slow down. Intermittent fasting can influence metabolic rate, and some women may find their bodies adapting to the new eating pattern. Adjusting the fasting window or incorporating specific foods can help counteract this.

3. **3. Social Pressures:** The social aspect of eating plays a significant role in our lives, and societal norms often revolve around

traditional meal times. Overcoming the pressure to conform to these norms while practicing intermittent fasting requires both self-assurance and effective communication with friends and family.

Strategies for Long-Term Success:

Now, let's delve into effective strategies to ensure not just short-term gains but long-term success in your intermittent fasting journey.

1. **Gradual Transition:** Rome wasn't built in a day, and your fasting routine need not be either. Consider a gradual transition, allowing your body to adapt at its own pace. Start with a 12-hour fasting window and slowly extend it based on your comfort level.

2. **Tailored Approaches:** Recognize that one size does not fit all. Customizing your intermittent fasting plan to align with your lifestyle, preferences, and health needs is crucial. Whether it's the 16/8 method or alternate-day fasting, find what suits you best.

3. **Nutrient-Rich Foods:** Focus on nutrient-dense meals to ensure you're meeting your body's requirements. Include a variety of fruits, vegetables, lean proteins, and whole grains in your eating window to promote overall health and well-being.

Mindful Eating (Portion Control) and Emotional Well-being:

Mindful eating is an integral aspect of intermittent fasting, promoting a healthy relationship with food and fostering emotional well-being.

1. **Portion Control:** Paying attention to portion sizes is fundamental. Even within the fasting window, it's essential to consume balanced, portion-controlled meals to meet nutritional needs without overindulging.

2. **Emotional Well-being:** Emotional eating can pose challenges during intermittent fasting. Develop mindfulness techniques to distinguish between physical hunger and emotional cues. Engage in activities that

bring joy and relaxation, reducing the reliance on food for emotional comfort.

Overcoming challenges and staying consistent with intermittent fasting is about embracing a holistic approach. It's not just about the clock; it's about nourishing your body, understanding its unique needs, and fostering a positive relationship with food. As a woman over 40, you have the wisdom and resilience to navigate this journey with grace, empowering yourself towards lasting health and vitality.

Conclusion

Congratulations on embarking on this transformative journey towards a healthier, more vibrant you. As we wrap up our exploration of intermittent fasting for women over 40, it's time to celebrate the strides you've made in mastering weight management, soothing stomach woes, and cultivating optimal gut wellness through the power of IF and delectable recipes.

Celebrating Your Health Journey:

Your commitment to intermittent fasting reflects a profound dedication to your well-being. Acknowledge and celebrate the milestones you've achieved on this path—whether it's shedding a few pounds, experiencing increased energy levels, or finding a sense of balance in your relationship with food. Each step forward is a victory worth commemorating.

Remember that health is not solely measured by the number on a scale but by the vitality and strength you feel within. Embrace the small victories, relish the positive changes, and take pride in the intentional choices you've made to nurture your body.

Looking Ahead to a Vibrant Future:

As you reflect on the incredible journey so far, cast your gaze toward a future filled with vitality and well-being. Intermittent fasting is not just a temporary fix; it's a sustainable lifestyle that can continue to enrich your health in the years to come.

Consider how you can further enhance your wellness journey. Perhaps there are new recipes you'd like to try, different fasting windows to experiment with, or additional mindful practices to incorporate into your routine. The future is a canvas waiting for your brushstrokes, and your health is a masterpiece in the making.

Continue to prioritize self-care, savor the nourishment of wholesome foods, and cherish the moments of mindfulness that intermittent fasting has brought into your life. This journey is ongoing, and each day presents an opportunity to embrace well-being with open arms.

In closing, know that you are not alone in this pursuit. Countless women over 40 share similar aspirations, challenges, and triumphs. Your commitment to intermittent fasting is a testament to your resilience and the value you place on living a healthy, fulfilling life.

May your path be illuminated by the radiance of good health, and may you continue to savour the journey towards a vibrant future. Cheers to you and the remarkable woman you are becoming through the art of intermittent fasting!

Bonus: 28-Day Meal Planner Journal

Guide to Using Your 28-Day Meal Planner Journal

Date and Day:

- Begin by entering the specific date and day of the week at the top of the page. This helps you keep track of your progress throughout the 28-day journey.

Fasting Window:

- Note the start and end times of your fasting window for the day. This is the period during which you abstain from consuming calories.

Meal Sections:

- Breakfast, Lunch, Dinner:

- List the foods you plan to eat for each meal. Include portion sizes to maintain mindful eating habits.

- Snacks:

- Record any snacks you consume between meals.

Hydration:

- Keep track of your water intake throughout the day. Staying hydrated is essential for overall well-being.

Exercise:

- If applicable, log your physical activity for the day. This can include workouts, walks, or any form of exercise you engage in.

Notes/Reflections:

- Use this space to jot down any thoughts or reflections related to your meals. Consider noting how certain foods make you feel or any challenges you encountered.

Remember, this journal is a tool to enhance your intermittent fasting journey. Personalize it to suit your preferences, and use it as a guide to cultivate healthier habits over the next 28 days.

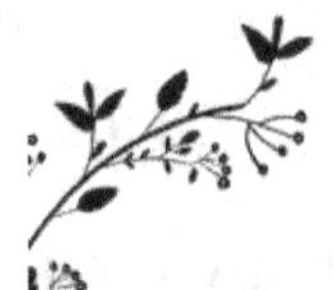 

DAILY MEAL PLANNER

DATE AND DAY:

BREAKFAST

FASTING WINDOW

START:

STOP:

LUNCH

EXCERCISES

DINNER

NOTES

SNACKS

HYDRATION

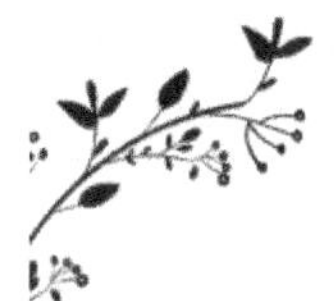# DAILY MEAL PLANNER 

DATE AND DAY:

M T W T F S S

BREAKFAST

FASTING WINDOW

START:

STOP:

LUNCH

EXCERCISES

○
○
○
○

DINNER

NOTES

SNACKS

HYDRATION

○
○
○

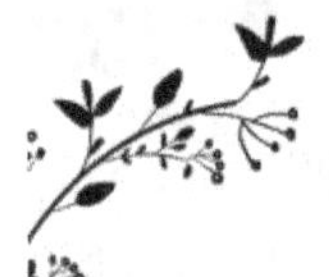 # DAILY MEAL PLANNER 

DATE AND DAY:

M T W T F S S

BREAKFAST

FASTING WINDOW

START: ___________________

STOP: ___________________

LUNCH

EXCERCISES

○ ___________________
○ ___________________
○ ___________________
○ ___________________

DINNER

NOTES

SNACKS

HYDRATION

○ ___________________
○ ___________________
○ ___________________

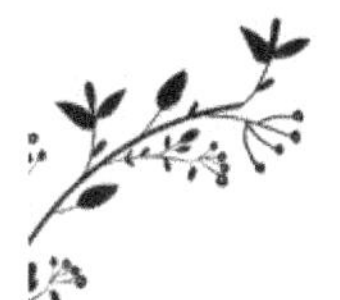

DAILY MEAL PLANNER

DATE AND DAY:

M T W T F S S

....

BREAKFAST

FASTING WINDOW

START: ______________________

STOP: ______________________

LUNCH

EXCERCISES

- ○ ____________________
- ○ ____________________
- ○ ____________________
- ○ ____________________

DINNER

NOTES

SNACKS

HYDRATION

- ○ ____________________
- ○ ____________________
- ○ ____________________

DAILY MEAL PLANNER

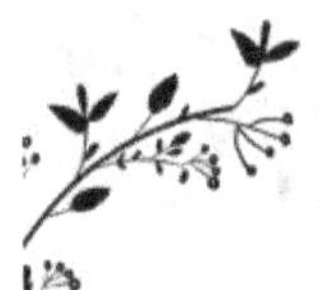

DATE AND DAY:

M T W T F S S

....

BREAKFAST

FASTING WINDOW

START: ___________________

STOP: ___________________

LUNCH

EXCERCISES

- ___________________
- ___________________
- ___________________
- ___________________

DINNER

NOTES

SNACKS

HYDRATION

- ___________________
- ___________________
- ___________________

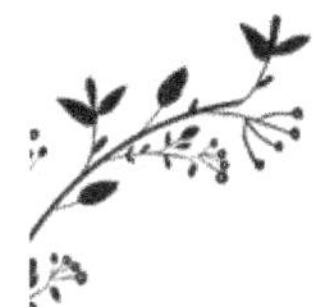 

DAILY MEAL PLANNER

DATE AND DAY:

M T W T F S S

BREAKFAST

LUNCH

DINNER

SNACKS

HYDRATION

FASTING WINDOW

START:

STOP:

EXCERCISES

NOTES

DAILY MEAL PLANNER

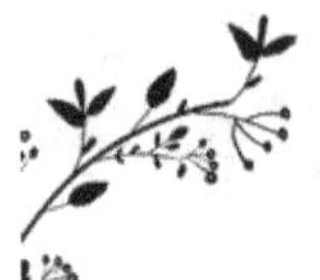

DATE AND DAY:

M T W T F S S

....

BREAKFAST

LUNCH

DINNER

SNACKS

HYDRATION

○ ______________________
○ ______________________
○ ______________________

FASTING WINDOW

START: ______________________

STOP: ______________________

EXCERCISES

○ ______________________
○ ______________________
○ ______________________
○ ______________________

NOTES

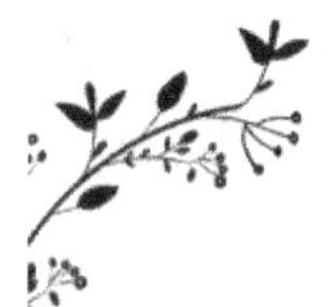 # DAILY MEAL PLANNER 

DATE AND DAY:

M T W T F S S

....

BREAKFAST

FASTING WINDOW

START: ______________________

STOP: ______________________

LUNCH

EXCERCISES

○ ______________________
○ ______________________
○ ______________________
○ ______________________

DINNER

NOTES

SNACKS

HYDRATION

○ ______________________
○ ______________________
○ ______________________

DAILY MEAL PLANNER

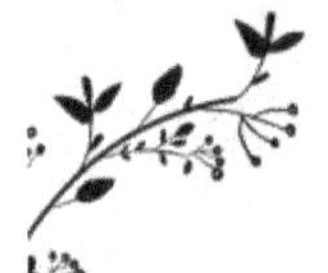

DATE AND DAY:

M T W T F S S

BREAKFAST

LUNCH

DINNER

SNACKS

HYDRATION

FASTING WINDOW

START:

STOP:

EXCERCISES

NOTES

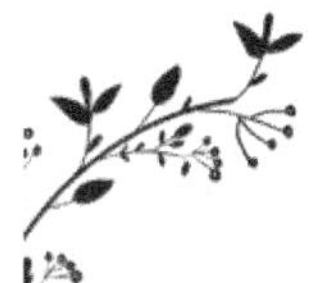

DAILY MEAL PLANNER

DATE AND DAY:

M T W T F S S

....

BREAKFAST

FASTING WINDOW

START: _______________

STOP: _______________

LUNCH

EXCERCISES

○ _______________
○ _______________
○ _______________
○ _______________

DINNER

NOTES

SNACKS

HYDRATION

○ _______________
○ _______________
○ _______________

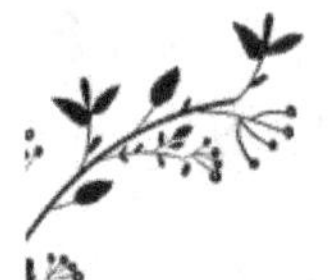 

DAILY MEAL PLANNER

DATE AND DAY:

M T W T F S S

BREAKFAST

FASTING WINDOW

START: ___________________

STOP: ___________________

LUNCH

EXCERCISES

○ ___________________
○ ___________________
○ ___________________
○ ___________________

DINNER

NOTES

SNACKS

HYDRATION

○ ___________________
○ ___________________
○ ___________________

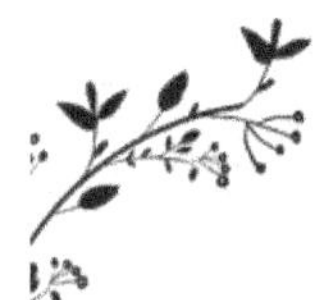 

DAILY MEAL PLANNER

DATE AND DAY:

M T W T F S S

BREAKFAST

LUNCH

DINNER

SNACKS

HYDRATION

FASTING WINDOW

START:

STOP:

EXCERCISES

NOTES

DAILY MEAL PLANNER

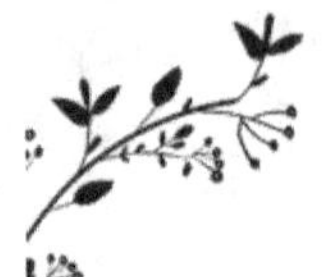 

DATE AND DAY:

M T W T F S S

....

BREAKFAST

FASTING WINDOW

START: _______________

STOP: _______________

LUNCH

EXCERCISES

○ _______________
○ _______________
○ _______________
○ _______________

DINNER

NOTES

SNACKS

HYDRATION

○ _______________
○ _______________
○ _______________

DAILY MEAL PLANNER

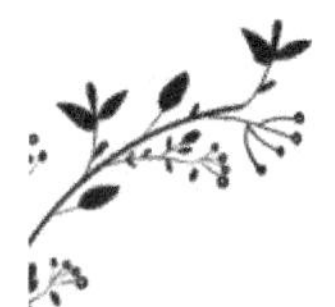

DATE AND DAY:

M T W T F S S

BREAKFAST

LUNCH

DINNER

SNACKS

HYDRATION

FASTING WINDOW

START:

STOP:

EXCERCISES

NOTES

DAILY MEAL PLANNER

DATE AND DAY:

M T W T F S S

BREAKFAST

FASTING WINDOW

START: ______________

STOP: ______________

LUNCH

EXCERCISES

- ○ ______________
- ○ ______________
- ○ ______________
- ○ ______________

DINNER

NOTES

SNACKS

HYDRATION

- ○ ______________
- ○ ______________
- ○ ______________

DAILY MEAL PLANNER

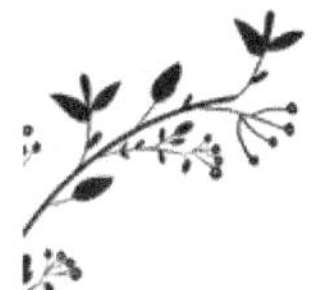
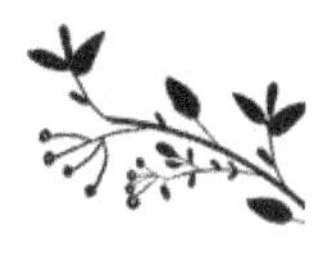

DATE AND DAY:

M T W T F S S

....

BREAKFAST

FASTING WINDOW

START: ______________________

STOP: ______________________

LUNCH

EXCERCISES

○ ______________________
○ ______________________
○ ______________________
○ ______________________

DINNER

NOTES

SNACKS

HYDRATION

○ ______________________
○ ______________________
○ ______________________

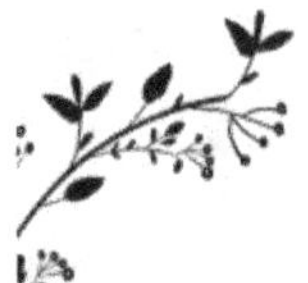 # DAILY MEAL PLANNER 

DATE AND DAY:

M T W T F S S

BREAKFAST

FASTING WINDOW

START: ______________________

STOP: ______________________

LUNCH

EXCERCISES

○ ______________________
○ ______________________
○ ______________________
○ ______________________

DINNER

NOTES

SNACKS

HYDRATION

○ ______________________
○ ______________________
○ ______________________

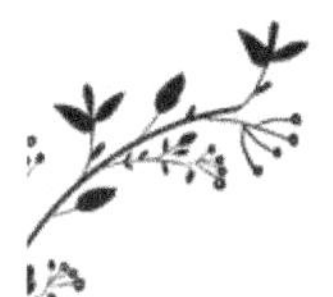# DAILY MEAL PLANNER 

DATE AND DAY:

M T W T F S S

BREAKFAST

FASTING WINDOW

START:

STOP:

LUNCH

EXCERCISES

DINNER

NOTES

SNACKS

HYDRATION

DAILY MEAL PLANNER

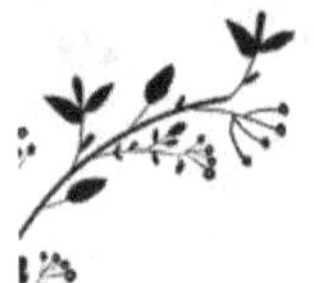

DATE AND DAY:

M T W T F S S

....

BREAKFAST

FASTING WINDOW

START: __________________

STOP: __________________

LUNCH

EXCERCISES

- ○ __________________
- ○ __________________
- ○ __________________
- ○ __________________

DINNER

NOTES

SNACKS

HYDRATION

- ○ __________________
- ○ __________________
- ○ __________________

DAILY MEAL PLANNER

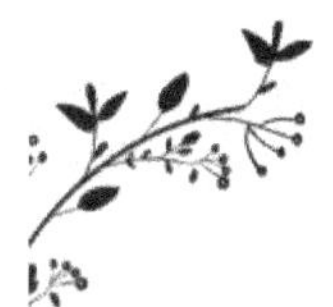

DATE AND DAY:

BREAKFAST

LUNCH

DINNER

SNACKS

HYDRATION

FASTING WINDOW

START:

STOP:

EXCERCISES

NOTES

DAILY MEAL PLANNER

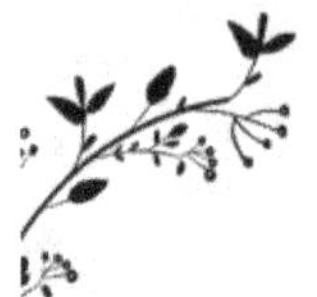

DATE AND DAY:

M T W T F S S

....

BREAKFAST

FASTING WINDOW

START: ______________________

STOP: ______________________

LUNCH

EXCERCISES

- ◯ ______________________
- ◯ ______________________
- ◯ ______________________
- ◯ ______________________

DINNER

NOTES

SNACKS

HYDRATION

- ◯ ______________________
- ◯ ______________________
- ◯ ______________________

DAILY MEAL PLANNER

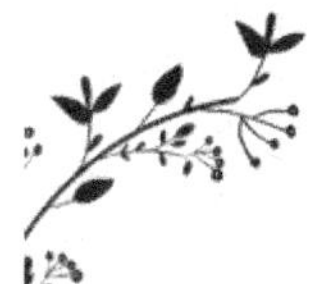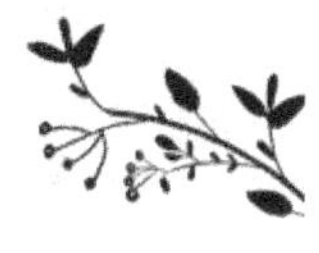

DATE AND DAY:

M T W T F S S

....

BREAKFAST

FASTING WINDOW

START: _______________

STOP: _______________

LUNCH

EXCERCISES

○ _______________
○ _______________
○ _______________
○ _______________

DINNER

NOTES

SNACKS

HYDRATION

○ _______________
○ _______________
○ _______________

DAILY MEAL PLANNER

DATE AND DAY:

M T W T F S S

BREAKFAST

FASTING WINDOW

START: _______________

STOP: _______________

LUNCH

EXCERCISES

○ _______________
○ _______________
○ _______________
○ _______________

DINNER

NOTES

SNACKS

HYDRATION

○ _______________
○ _______________
○ _______________

DAILY MEAL PLANNER

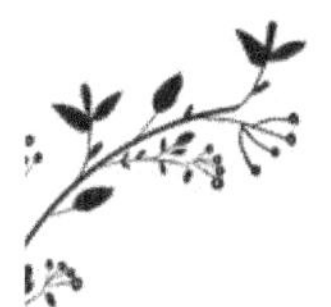

DATE AND DAY:

....

M T W T F S S

BREAKFAST

LUNCH

DINNER

SNACKS

HYDRATION

○ ________________________________
○ ________________________________
○ ________________________________

FASTING WINDOW

START: ________________________

STOP: ________________________

EXERCISES

○ ________________________________
○ ________________________________
○ ________________________________
○ ________________________________

NOTES

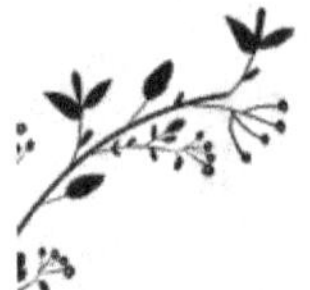 

DAILY MEAL PLANNER

DATE AND DAY:

M T W T F S S

BREAKFAST

LUNCH

DINNER

SNACKS

HYDRATION

FASTING WINDOW

START: _______________

STOP: _______________

EXCERCISES

NOTES

DAILY MEAL PLANNER

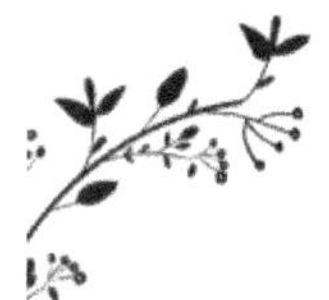

DATE AND DAY:

M T W T F S S

BREAKFAST

FASTING WINDOW

START: ___________________

STOP: ___________________

LUNCH

EXCERCISES

- ○ ___________________
- ○ ___________________
- ○ ___________________
- ○ ___________________

DINNER

NOTES

SNACKS

HYDRATION

- ○ ___________________
- ○ ___________________
- ○ ___________________

DAILY MEAL PLANNER

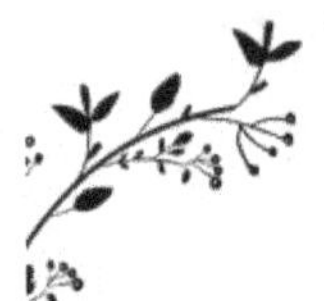

DATE AND DAY:

M T W T F S S

BREAKFAST

LUNCH

DINNER

SNACKS

HYDRATION

FASTING WINDOW

START:

STOP:

EXCERCISES

NOTES

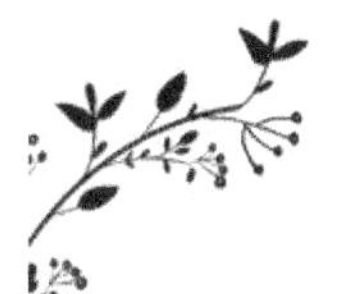 # DAILY MEAL PLANNER 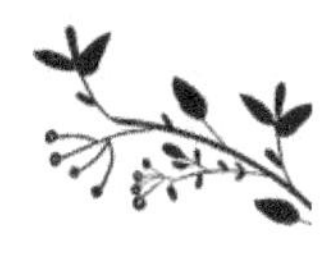

DATE AND DAY:

M T W T F S S

....

BREAKFAST

FASTING WINDOW

START: ______________________

STOP: ______________________

LUNCH

EXCERCISES

○ ______________________
○ ______________________
○ ______________________
○ ______________________

DINNER

NOTES

SNACKS

HYDRATION

○ ______________________
○ ______________________
○ ______________________

Thanks for reading

Dear Reader,

As you close the final chapter of "Intermittent Fasting for Women Over 40," we extend our heartfelt gratitude for allowing us to be part of your health and wellness exploration. Your commitment to these pages reflects a shared pursuit—to embrace the vitality that comes with mastering intermittent fasting.

Remember, this isn't the end; it's a new beginning. Your newfound wisdom on weight management, stomach wellness, and gut health will undoubtedly become valuable tools in your daily life. May the strategies for overcoming challenges and staying consistent serve as beacons on your path to long-term success.

As you close the cover, we want you to carry with you the assurance that this book is not merely a collection of words—it's a testament to your strength, resilience, and commitment to your well-being.

Thank you for entrusting us with a small part of your journey. May you continue to thrive, finding joy in each step, and savouring the delectable flavours of a life well-lived.

With sincere appreciation,

Dr Marcia Moss

Mail: drmarciamoss@gmail.com